Healing from a Grace Perspective

Live and Not Die

Don't live with Chronic Pain or Disease

Sonja H. Parham

ISBN 978-1-0980-2062-0 (paperback)
ISBN 978-1-0980-2063-7 (digital)

Christian Faith Publishing, Inc.
832 Park Avenue
Meadville, PA 16335
www.christianfaithpublishing.com

Printed in the United States of America

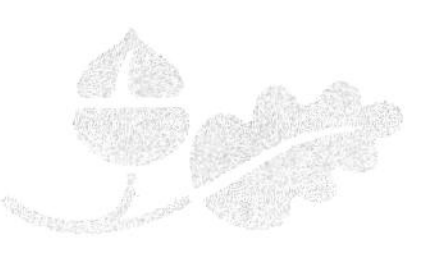

Contents

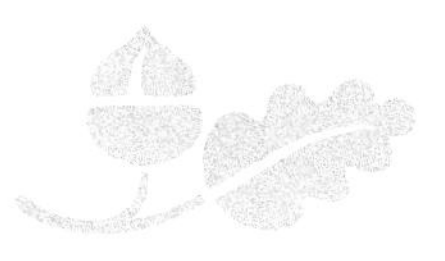

INTRODUCTION

This book was written for the purpose of helping you to understand the power of the Word of God in destroying sickness and disease and to teach you how to apply the Word of God by faith to take the healing that belongs to you as a born-again believer. If you have not accepted Jesus as your Lord and Savior go to the back cover of this book and say the sinner's prayer with all your heart and you will be saved.

If you have accepted Jesus as your personal Lord and Savior, then healing belongs to you. It doesn't matter if you are being attacked by Satan with cancer, chronic pain, heart disease, the Word of God has enough power in it to destroy *all* manner of sickness and *all* manner of disease when applied with precision.

Let's define *divine healing* as healing by the power of the Holy Spirit or healing by standing on the Word of God. It's healing beyond man-made methods. It's supernatural healing.

This book will teach you divine healing from a grace perspective. You may ask, "What does that mean?"

Grace is God's undeserved and unmerited favor. God, by his grace (God's undeserved favor), has already released his healing power for every man that will ever need healing. Healing is on the inside of you if you are born again. God gave you healing by His grace (God's undeserved favor) not because you earned it or deserved it, but he just favored you and gave it to you as a gift. Grace has made healing available, but you must respond with your faith to take it. The kingdom of God is on the inside of you, and that kingdom has healing in it.

If you are born again, then you have a covenant with God through Jesus Christ, and that covenant has healing in it. Let's define a covenant.

A *covenant* is an agreement initiated by God with well-defined terms and sealed with an oath for delivery. The Scriptures in the New Testament are the well-defined terms of the grace covenant that you are in. Whatever God has already said in the Scriptures can't be changed and are established laws of the covenant.

Healing is your covenant right as a believer. Remember, Jesus was talking to the religious leaders of his day and said, "And ought not this woman, being a daughter of Abraham, whom Satan hath bound, lo, these eighteen years, be loosed from this bond on the sabbath day" (Luke 13:16, KJV).

This woman was a Jew and was in covenant with God; therefore, Jesus said she should be healed because healing belonged to her in the covenant.

Even in the old covenant of the Law (Ten Commandments), Jesus recognized that the woman was entitled to healing because she was a Jew in covenant with God. Much more as a born-again believer today, you are entitled to healing because healing is in the atonement of Jesus Christ. This means Jesus purchased your healing two thousand years ago, long before you would ever need it. Healing belongs to you under the new covenant of grace. Jesus has paid for your healing with the thirty-nine stripes that he took on his back. You are in covenant with God through Jesus Christ, and the Scriptures in the New Testament are the well-defined terms of that covenant. Grace (God's undeserved favor) has made healing available to you, but you must take what grace (God's undeserved favor) has made available by faith. Grace always require a response, and that response is called faith. So we can now define faith as "our positive response to what grace has made available."

When there is a part of your life that is not reflecting the covenant and the things of the covenant, such as healing, prosperity, wholeness, soundness, and all the finished works of Jesus Christ, then you are living below your covenant rights. This is called a substandard life, where you are not living the full potential of the covenant that

Jesus died for you to have. God never intended for his children to live substandard lives in any area; however, so many Christians are living below God's standard and below their covenant rights, especially in the area of healing and finances. They don't receive what God has already done for them through Jesus and what he has already said in his Word because of religion, tradition of men, and not having knowledge of their covenant. One of the well-defined terms of the covenant says, "Who his own self bare our sins in his own body on the tree, that we, being dead to sins, should live unto righteousness: by whose stripes ye *were healed*" (1 Pet. 2:24) so healing belongs to you.

A great deal of Christians today don't know anything about their covenant and how to access the covenant for healing. Our lack of knowledge is causing us to perish with sickness and disease, especially from the fowl spirit of *cancer*. The Bible says, "My people are destroyed for lack of knowledge" (Hosea 4:6).

Satan destroys us when we don't know about our covenant and the kingdom of God and how to get the kingdom to produce what we need in our lives. The Bible says, "The thief cometh not, but *for* to steal, and to kill, and to destroy: I am come that they might have life, and that they might have it more abundantly" (John 10:10). This Scripture is in red print in the Bible, which means this is actually Jesus talking, and he says that Satan is the one that kills, steal, and destroy. Notice the Scripture says that Jesus is the one that came to bring life and bring it more abundantly.

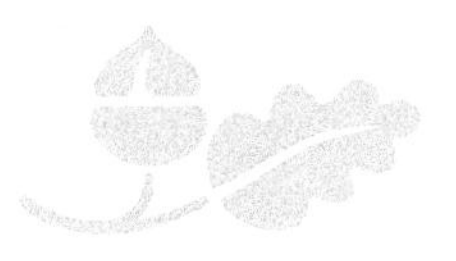

Grace Has Made Healing Available

If you have received Jesus Christ as your Lord and Savior, you already have everything you will ever need in this life on the inside of you. Everything that God has given you, he has given it to you through Jesus as an act of his grace (God's undeserved favor). God does everything by *grace*!

Let's define grace as God doing for you independent of you. Grace is God's undeserved favor. Grace is God releasing his power and ability on your behalf. Grace is Jesus! God's grace (God's undeserved favor) is the same toward every man. You don't deserve anything from God, and you certainly couldn't earn anything from Him. God by his grace (God's undeserved favor) has given you everything you will ever need in this life to include healing. He has given you everything through Jesus because he loves you and He is good. The Bible says, "He that spared not his own Son, but delivered him up for us all, how shall he not with him also freely give us all things" (Rom. 8:32, KJV)?

God poured his grace out for healing two thousand years ago for any man that would ever need healing. God poured his grace out for healing before you ever had a problem. The Bible says, "For the law was given by Moses, but grace and truth came by Jesus Christ" (John 1:17, KJV).

Grace came by Jesus and the law (Ten Commandments) came by Moses. On the cross at Calvary, Jesus established a new covenant with God the Father, and that covenant is called grace. If you have received Jesus Christ as your Lord and Savior, you are under the covenant of grace not the law (Ten Commandments), which is a performance-based covenant.

The grace covenant has salvation in it and the word *salvation* is translated in the Greek as "SOZO," which implies forgiveness of sins, healing, deliverance, perseverance, prosperity, and wholeness. Your salvation is more than just forgiveness of sins, but it is also includes healing. God, by his grace (God's undeserved favor), released his healing power through Jesus over two thousand years ago just for you. God, by his grace (God's undeserved favor), has provided healing, and when you accepted Jesus Christ as your Lord and Savior, healing was given to you. Well, you may ask if that is true, then why aren't every Christian healed. Every Christian isn't healed because you have to respond to what grace has made available through faith. The Bible says, "Through whom also *we have access by faith into this grace* in which we stand, and rejoice in hope of the glory of God" (Rom. 5:2, NKJV).

Grace is God's part but faith is your part. Although God, by his grace, has made healing available to you that healing has to be taken by faith. Remember, God had given the children of Israel Canaan land. It belonged to them, but they had to possess it. Grace has given you healing but you must possess it.

You must believe in grace, you must believe that healing has already been provided. You are not trying to get God to make healing for you. You are not trying to get God to heal you. Healing is a finished work of Jesus Christ. God, by his grace (God's undeserved favor), has released healing power to you through Jesus Christ. You must believe this!

You are not fighting from a place of defeat, but you are fighting from a place of victory that Jesus obtained for you two thousand years ago. You are not trying to get healed, but you are protecting the healing Jesus gave you two thousand years ago, and Satan is trying to steal it. The Bible says, "The thief cometh not, but for to steal, and to kill, and to destroy: I am come that they might have life, and that they might have it more abundantly" (John 10:10, KJV).

Jesus says in this Scripture that Satan is the one that is killing, stealing, and destroying. But notice Jesus also said he came to give life abundantly. Satan is trying to steal your healing.

You have been given the same power that raised Jesus from the dead on the inside of you. It's in your spirit. Healing is already on the inside of you in your spirit! You are displaying symptoms of sickness in your physical body, but the spirit man that lives on the inside of you is not sick.

If you can understand grace and how God has given you everything by his grace (God's undeserved favor) and that you didn't get it by your good deeds or performance and that you didn't earn anything, then you would recognize that healing is a gift to you from Jesus, and it's on the inside of you, and it can manifest on your physical body.

Most Christians have trouble believing that everything is already done because of religion and tradition of men have taught that you have to do so many good deeds in order for God to bless you or to receive healing. Religion has taught that if you are not living right, then God won't bless you. Do you realize that everyone that was healed in the Bible by Jesus was a sinner? It's not individual sins that make you a sinner in the eyes of God, but it's a sin nature that makes you a sinner in the eyes of God. All the people in Jesus's day had a sin nature because Jesus hadn't gone to the cross or died for man to be born again with a righteous nature. They were sinners and Jesus still healed them. That's the grace of God!

So just like in Jesus's day, sin didn't keep the people from receiving their healing, sin will not keep you from receiving your healing. This is the grace of God! Now let me say that I don't condone sin, stay out of sin because sin gives the devil authority to enter into your life and bring his destruction. The Bible says,

> And the prayer of faith shall save the sick, and the Lord shall raise him up; and if he have committed sins, they shall be forgiven him. *Confess your faults one to another,* and pray one for another, that ye may be healed. The effectual

> fervent prayer of a righteous man availeth much.
> (James 5:15–16, KJV)

Why does this Scripture say, "confess your faults one to another" in an effort to be healed? Because if you confess your faults, then you can be told that God is not holding those faults against you. In other words, some people may think, "I won't receive my healing because of something I did in the past." The Bible says confess those faults and receive God's grace of forgiveness.

Religion teaches that you have to do something to get God to do something. That God responds to man based on his performance. Under the old covenant of the law, God was responding to man based on his performance. That covenant was a performance-based covenant. If you did good and not sin, you got the blessing from God; but if you sinned, you got the curse. We are not under a performance-based covenant today but a grace-based covenant where God is being good to you not based on your behavior or performance but is solely based on what Jesus has done for you. Under this covenant of grace, you simply believe, receive and say thank you.

To further explain how grace works, let's look at how you received your salvation because how you receive salvation is how you receive your healing.

The Bible says, "For the grace of God that brings salvation has appeared to all men" (Titus 2:11, NKJV).

Grace (*God's undeserved favor*) has made salvation available to all men. God released his power for every man to receive salvation two thousand years ago through Jesus. If God's grace has made salvation available to all men, why aren't all men saved? All men are not saved because all men have not released faith for salvation although grace has made it available to them.

The Bible says, "Blessed be the God and Father of our Lord Jesus Christ, who *hath* blessed us with all spiritual blessings in heavenly places in Christ" (Eph. 1:3, KJV). Healing is a spiritual blessing; therefore, healing is on the inside of you. The word *hath* is past tense. God, by his grace, has already blessed you with the spiritual blessing of healing.

If you believe and understand that God, by his grace (God's undeserved favor), has made healing available to you, then you will recognize that there is nothing left for God to do.

Grace makes but faith takes! You must understand that you have a covenant with God through Jesus Christ, and that healing is in that covenant. You must renew your mind to the fact that healing is on the inside of you and release your faith for your healing. We will discuss how to do that further in this book. You must believe that healing exist on the inside of you. The Bible says, "that the sharing of your faith may become effective *by the acknowledgment of every good thing which is in you in Christ Jesus*" (Philem. 6, NKJV). The word *communicate* means "to release or transfer," and the word *effectual* means "to begin to work or produce." The word *acknowledge* means "to admit to the existence of a thing." Therefore, this Scripture clearly states that your faith starts to release and begin to work or produce when you acknowledge and admit that healing is on the inside of you. Grace has made healing available!

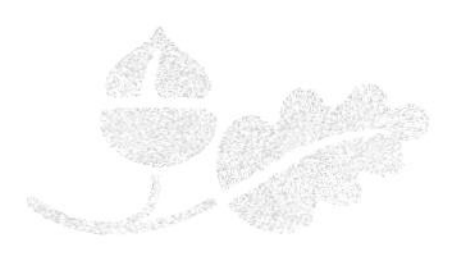

Healing is in Your Covenant

If you are experiencing symptoms of sickness in your body, the disease that is trying to destroy you is from Satan, but Jesus has come that you *may* have life and have it more abundantly. Notice the Scripture says you "may" have life and have it more abundantly. Having the abundant life is conditional. Having the abundant life is not automatic, it depends on how much you understand the kingdom of God and how to get the kingdom of God to manifest what has already been given to you by Jesus Christ. Whether you receive that abundant life is going to depend on how well you understand your covenant of grace and how well you operate in the principles and the laws that govern the kingdom of God.

The Bible teaches that there are several ways in which you can be healed. The two primary ways of being divinely healed by God is through the laying on of hands and releasing faith in the Word of God. You can be healed by someone who has been anointed by God with healing power and is a carrier of that healing power. They can lay hands on you, and if you release your faith, that healing power will flow into your body and destroy the disease. But what if you don't have anyone in your area that is a carrier of God's healing power? You can be healed simply by believing and acting on the Word of God. This type of healing is called being healed by faith. This book will teach you the method of being healed by faith.

Even if no one lay hands on you or pray, you can take your healing by simply acting on the Word of God. There is no sickness or disease that can stand up against the power of the Word of God when the Word is applied appropriately with working knowledge. Jesus said he has given us the keys of the kingdom. "And *I will give you* the keys of the kingdom of heaven, and whatever you bind on earth will be bound in heaven, and whatever you loose on earth will be loosed in heaven" (Matt. 16:19).

The Kingdom operate by keys because the Bible says, "Woe to you lawyers! For you have taken away the key of knowledge. You did not enter in yourselves, and those who were entering in you hindered" (Luke 11:52).

One of the keys of the kingdom is knowledge, *revelation knowledge of God's Word.* Another key of the kingdom is understanding. When you get revelation knowledge and understanding of how God's Word operates, you can take from the kingdom whatever you need to include healing.

The knowledge, revelation, and understanding that you will receive from this book will enable you to act on the Word of God and take the healing that has already been provided by grace (God's undeserved favor).

As a Christian, you must understand that you have a covenant with God, and to receive from God, you must respond to him based on your covenant because God is a covenant-keeping God. You must be a covenant practitioner acting on the covenant. The Bible says, "My covenant will I not break, nor alter the thing that is gone out of my lips" (Ps. 89:34). This is God himself speaking.

God also says, "He hath remembered his covenant for ever, the word which he commanded to a thousand generations" (Ps. 105:8).

The Scriptures in the Bible (New Testament) is God's covenant promises, and what he says about your healing is already done, you just have to believe it and release your faith for it. When God says, "Who his own self bare our sins in his own body on the tree, that we, being dead to sins, should live unto righteousness: by whose stripes ye were healed" (1 Pet. 2:24). This is your covenant, and it belongs to you. The Scripture says you *were* (past tense) healed. You must now believe this and receive it by faith.

You have a right to healing because through Jesus, you have a covenant with God, and healing is in that covenant. You can therefore say, "God, I have a right to be healed because Jesus purchased my healing two thousand years ago with the stripes he bore on his back, and I am in covenant with you through Jesus."

This covenant of grace that has provided healing now makes all the unscriptural things that you have heard, such as: "God heals people in his own time" is not true. God provided healing for every man two thousand years ago, and if you are in the covenant of grace through Jesus, healing belongs to you. Another saying that is unscriptural is "It's not God's will to heal everybody," this is not true because God released his healing power through Jesus two thousand years ago, and it's just a matter of Christians knowing about their covenant of grace and receiving what has been provided for them. In these last days, there are two things that Christians must know, and that is who they are and what belongs to them.

God's grace is the same to all men, and God is no respecter of person. This now takes the responsibility off God for your healing and put it on you. If you are wondering if God will heal you, that should not be a question for you because you now know that God has already provided the healing, all you have to do is take it. Knowing your covenant of grace makes life so much easier. Jesus said, "Take my yoke upon you, and learn of me; for I am meek and lowly in heart: and ye shall find rest unto your souls" (Matt. 11:29).

Christian people should not be struggling to receive from God because God has made everything available to include healing through grace (Jesus). Once we learn of the covenant of grace and what belongs to us, we just simply have to know how to receive it. Grace has made healing available to you, but you must take it by faith.

In conclusion, I want you to know and understand by grace (*the unearned, undeserved favor of God*) has already healed every man that will ever need healing. Healing was made available by grace (*the unearned, undeserved favor of God*) two thousand years ago. You are not trying to get God to heal you, but you are simply maintaining the healing that Jesus provided for you two thousand years ago. Satan is trying to take the healing that Jesus has already given you. Therefore, you must understand that you are fighting from a place of victory, not a place of defeat. You are not asking God to heal you, but rather, you are maintaining the healing that Jesus has already given you.

God, by his grace (*the unearned, undeserved favor of God*), has made healing available to every man that will ever need it. The Bible says, "Blessed be the God and Father of our Lord Jesus Christ, *who has blessed us with* every spiritual blessing in the heavenly places in Christ" (Eph. 1:3). Healing is a spiritual blessing. You might be saying, "Well, if I have healing, then where is it?" It's in the spirit part of you. It's in Christ and he is on the inside of you. To locate healing and to get it to manifest, you must understand spirit, soul, and body.

Before going any further, please say this prayer with all your heart aloud.

> Father,
>
> I thank you that two thousand years ago, Jesus obtained my healing for me on the whipping post; however, Satan is trying to take it. I believe according to *1 Peter 2:24* that by Jesus's stripes, I am already healed. That healing is in the spirit part of me, and I must bring it into the physical realm where I can experience it on my physical body. This book will provide instruction as to how to pull the healing out of the spirit realm into the physical realm. I ask that you give me clear understanding, revelation knowledge, and wisdom of the instructions in this book. Holy Spirit, help me to be quick to believe and not doubt what I read in this book. Help me to act on what I read and see in this book for I know that acting on the Word will produce results. I thank you, Father, for providing this book so I can take my healing. In Jesus's name, amen.

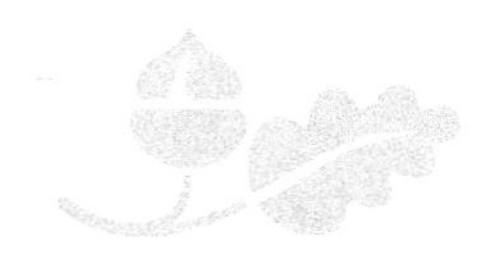

Spirit, Soul, and Body

Understanding sprit, soul, and body is essential in obtaining your healing. If I asked you to describe yourself to me, you would probably tell me your height, eye color, hair color, skin color, and weight. You would do this because you identify with your physical man as who you are. But the truth is, the real you is a spirit. You have a spirit man living on the inside of you who is the real you. In our daily life, we don't identify with the spirit man on the inside of us. We look at our behavior, thoughts, and actions to determine whether we are worthy of the blessings of God when the truth is, God does not use these external things to determine his goodness toward us because under the new covenant of grace (New Testament), God looks at us through our position in Christ and who we are in him. Understanding the functionality of spirit, soul, and body will forever change the way you relate to God and how you receive from him to include your healing.

You must understand that you are made of three parts. You are a spirit, you have a soul, and you live in a physical body. Religion has taught that the spirit and the soul are the same but they are not. They are different because the Bible says, "Now may the God of peace Himself sanctify you completely; and may your whole spirit, soul, and body be preserved blameless at the coming of our Lord Jesus Christ" (1 Thess. 5:23, NKJV). This Scripture differentiates between the spirit and the soul. We see by Scripture that they are not the same.

Your spirit is the real you, and your soul is your mind, will, emotions, personality, conscience. Your body is the house that your spirit and soul live in, and the spirit possesses the soul (mind).

You have a man living on the inside of you, and that man is called the spirit man or inner man. The spirit man was infected with sin because of Adam's sin in the garden of Eden. Therefore, every man born after Adam is born with that sin nature. This sin nature man kept you from fellowshipping with God, that's why Jesus had to come to give you a new righteousness nature man so you could fellowship with God and receive from him. The process of receiving this new righteous nature man that allows you to fellowship with God is called the new birth, where you are given a new spirit man on the inside of you and he is from heaven. The Bible says, "Therefore, if anyone is in Christ, he is a new creation; old things have passed away; behold, all things have become new" (2 Cor. 5:17, NKJV).

God put everything good to include healing in that new spirit man and then sealed your spirit with the Holy Spirit. The Bible says, "Blessed be the God and Father of our Lord Jesus Christ, who has blessed us with every spiritual blessing in the heavenly places in Christ" (Eph. 1:3, NKJV). Healing is a spiritual blessing! God did this by his grace (God's undeserved favor).

The Bible also says, "And that you put on the new man which was created according to God, in true righteousness and holiness" (Eph. 4:24, NKJV). You have been made righteous (right standing with God) and holy in your spirit. Your spirit is perfect and is just like Jesus.

You must understand that everything God gives you, he will give it to you in your spirit. Understanding your heart and how your heart works is vital in receiving healing. When the Bible speaks of the word *heart*, it's not talking about your physical heart that pumps blood, but it's talking about your reborn spirit and your soul (mind, will, emotions, conscience, attitudes, personality). *Your heart is made up of two parts*, the spirit and the soul (mind). One part of your heart is perfect, and that's the spirit but the soul (mind) is not perfect. The soul was not impacted by the new birth, only your spirit was made new according to (2 Cor. 5:17, NKJV). Therefore, your spirit believes all the things of God because your spirit is just like God, but it's your soul (mind) that doesn't believe the things of God. That is why the Bible says, "And be not conformed to this world: but be ye transformed by the renewing of your mind, that ye may prove what is that good, and acceptable, and perfect, will of God" (Rom. 12:2, KJV). To be conformed means to change.

You must change the way your mind currently thinks, where healing is concerned, and make it believe that healing is already on the inside of you. This is called renewing your mind with the word of God. To receive from God in any area of your life, your mind has to believe what the Word says in that area. A mind that doesn't believe the Word of God in any area is called the flesh. The flesh is a mindset contrary to the Word of God. It is vital to get your mind to believe what God has said in his Word about your healing. A mind that doesn't believe what God has said about your healing will fight against your spirit and hinder the spirit's ability to release that healing.

So healing is on the inside of you in your spirit. You must believe that healing already exist on the inside of you.

Your spirit believe the things of God because your spirit is from heaven if you are born-again, however, your mind has been trained by the world to believe contrary to the word of God. For example, your mind maybe struggling to believe what you are reading in this book but your spirit believe it and know that what you are reading is true. Your born-again spirit will bear witness with spiritual truth. You might have to read this book several times to get faith to come to you where this book is concern. As you read this book over and over again you will start to believe it.

Everything God gives you he give it to you in your spirit not your physical body. The bible says "the spirit of a man is the lamp of the lord (proverbs 20:27). God enlightens and give revelation to you in your spirit. Sickness and disease is on your physical body but is not in your spirit. Healing is in the spirit part of you. Understanding Spirit, Soul and Body is so important. Healing starts in your spirit the moment you pray".

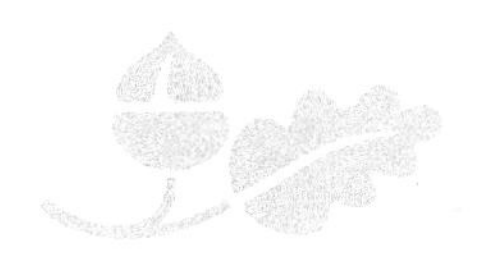

You Must Know that God Wants You Well

So many Christians today believe that God wants them saved. They have no questions where salvation is concern, but when it comes to healing, they question whether it's God's will to heal. They wonder if it is God's will to heal them. We hear sayings like: "God don't heal everybody, or healing is not for today." These saying are contrary to the Scriptures. The reason for this is because we've heard so much preaching and teaching on salvation, forgiveness of sins, being born again, but we haven't heard much preaching or teaching on healing. The Scriptures are spiritual laws that cannot be broken, and they operate in the kingdom of God. One of the spiritual laws of the kingdom of God is "So then faith comes by hearing, and hearing by the word of God" (Rom. 10:17, NKJV).

You can't have faith for something you have not heard. This is spiritual law. Knowledge always come before faith. You can't have faith for that which you have no knowledge. There has been very little teaching on divine healing from the Bible, and because of this, there isn't much faith for healing in the church today.

To give you an example of what I am saying, if I said to you, "You are not saved," you would probably get upset with me and say, "I am saved because I have accepted Jesus as Lord and Savior and been water baptized." It is unlikely that I could change your mind about your salvation. Well, the reason you could be so confident in your salvation is because you have heard so much about salvation through the preaching and teaching of the Word that you have a lot of faith in the new birth process and you receiving that new birth. However, if I said to you, "You are already healed," you probably would have great difficulty in believing that because of the symptoms that you are now experiencing in your body. Another reason you would struggle in believing you are already healed and healing is on the inside you is because you haven't heard much teaching and preaching on healing; therefore, there is no faith for healing. This is a real problem in the church today. So, let's look at healing from a grace perspective. Healing from a grace perspective means that healing is already done, it is a finished work of Jesus Christ. God is not going to make healing because you need it, God released his healing power for every man that would ever need it over two thousand years ago through Jesus and his finished works on the cross.

According to the Bible, Jesus purchased your healing and forgiveness of sins at the exact same time. Forgiveness of sins and deliverance from sickness and disease happened simultaneously and they can't be separated. Jesus see sin and sickness as the same. The Bible says, "Surely He has borne our griefs And carried our sorrows; Yet we esteemed Him stricken, Smitten by God, and afflicted. But He was wounded for our transgressions, He was bruised for our iniquities; The chastisement for our peace was upon Him, And by His stripes we are healed" (Isa. 53:4–5, NKJV) .

This is the plan of redemption and that plan was two-fold. To redeem means to buy back or to restore man back to his human dignity. Your redemption was twofold, forgiveness of sins and healing and you can't separate them. You notice the Scriptures says, "He was wounded for your transgressions," that word *transgressions* means "sin." Jesus took away your sins forever. But do you notice also that the same Scripture says, "And with His stripes you were healed." This is saying that Jesus healed you two thousand years ago with the thirty-nine stripes he took on his back and delivered you from sin all at the same time. Glory to God! So you can clearly see that forgiveness of sin and healing goes together, and they can't be separated. Forgiveness of sins and healing is in the atonement of our Lord and Savior, Jesus Christ. When I was studying this, the Lord said to me, "I dealt with healing first by taking that beating in Pilot's judgement hall, and then I dealt with sin on the cross. Healing was dealt with first."

What has happened is that religion has separated the two and teaches that your sins are forgiven by accepting Jesus as Lord and Savior but has said nothing about the other part of the plan of redemption, which is healing. Because of this, there is little or no faith for healing in much of the church today because faith can only come one way and that's by hearing (Romans 10:17). Let me say again, the plan of redemption was twofold, forgiveness of sins and healing, and they can't be separated. Healing belongs to you as a born-again believer. Healing is in the atonement of your Lord and Savior, Jesus Christ, and he died for your sickness just like he died for your sins at the same time. Glory to God! Now when you understand this, you will no longer consider all the religious things that people say such as "God don't heal everybody" or "healing is not for today." Jesus released his healing power by grace (God's undeserved favor) for every man that would every need healing two thousand years ago.

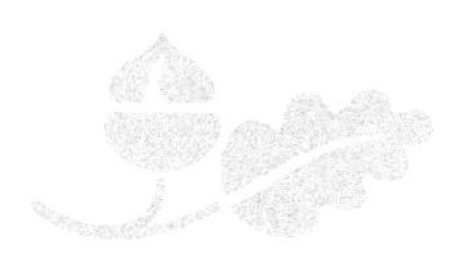

You Must Be Established in Righteousness

Let's define righteousness as "being in right standing with God." Before Jesus came, no man was in right standing with God because of sin (Adam's sin). Sin was a barrier that kept us separated from God. The Bible says,

> For he is our peace, who hath made both one, and hath broken down the middle wall of partition between us; Having abolished in his flesh the enmity, even the law of commandments contained in ordinances; for to make in himself of twain one new man, so making peace; And that he might reconcile both unto God in one body by the cross, having slain the enmity thereby. (Eph. 2: 14–16)

These Scriptures are saying that there was no peace between God and man because of Adam's sin. Man was separated from God as a middle wall of partition was between God and man. The word *enmity* means "feud." There was a feud between God and man because of sin, and there was no harmony. Verse 15 says that Jesus abolished the feud, combined the Jew and Gentile, and made one new man (the church). Jesus reconciled both the Jew and Gentile (church) to

God. Therefore, when you accepted Jesus as your Lord and Savior, you were put in right standing with God. God imputed righteousness into your spirit when you got born again. Remember, God gave you everything in your spirit. Your righteousness (right standing with God) is a gift. The Bible says, "For he hath made him to be sin for us, who knew no sin; that we might *be made* the righteousness of God in him" (2 Cor. 5:21).

This Scripture says that Jesus took all of your sins and became sin and gave you his righteousness. He made you righteous with God. Jesus put you in right standing with God. You didn't do anything to deserve righteousness, it was given to you as a gift. Under the covenant of grace, everything is done for you, and everything is a gift from Jesus. You don't have to do anything but believe and receive. You have to receive by faith! The Bible says, "For if by one man's offence death reigned by one; much more they which receive abundance of grace and of the *gift of righteousness* shall reign in life by one, Jesus Christ" (Rom. 5:17).

Notice the Scripture says that righteousness is a gift. Why is all of this so important? The reason why you must be established in righteousness is because *your righteousness (right standing with God) that Jesus gave you is the portal in which you receive everything from God.* Your position in Christ, which is righteousness, entitles you to all that Jesus has. All that Jesus has provided in the covenant of grace (healing, prosperity, deliverance, wholeness, soundness, salvation) belongs to you because of your right standing with God through Jesus. However, none of this will show up in your life until you release your faith for it. Remember what the Scripture says, "Who Himself bore our sins in His own body on the tree, that we, having died to sins, might live for righteousness—by whose stripes you were healed" (1 Pet. 2:24, NKJV). Notice this Scriptures says when we live to "righteousness," then by Jesus's stripes, we are healed. Healing comes to us through our righteousness. The righteousness that Jesus gave us.

You must understand that because you didn't do anything to earn righteousness (right standing with God), it's a gift to you that you can't sin your righteousness away. Religion teaches that once you sin, then you have to work toward getting back in right standing with God. This does not line up with the Scriptures. Under the covenant of grace, you didn't receive righteousness based on your performance or behavior, but you received it based on what Jesus did for you. Your sins (past, present, and future) were forgiven when Jesus died on the cross, and his (Jesus) righteousness was given to you when he was raised from the dead. Let's look at Scriptures that support what I just said. The Bible says, "This is the covenant that I will make with them after those days, saith the Lord, I will put my laws into their hearts, and in their minds will I write them; And their sins and iniquities will I remember no more" (Heb. 10:16).

In this Scripture, God himself is speaking. He is talking about the new covenant of grace that he is going to make with man through Jesus Christ after those days (after the days of Jesus resurrection). Under this new covenant of grace, God is saying that your sins he will remember no more. Your sins are forgiven (past, present, and future) under this new covenant of grace. Jesus paid the sin debt for you. The Bible says, "And he is the propitiation for our sins: and not for ours only, but also for the sins of the whole world" (1 John 2:2). This Scripture is talking about Jesus. The word *propitiation* means "payment (sin debt), ransom (deliverance from the law) and peace offering (between God and man)."

You being established in your righteousness is vital in receiving your healing. Sin is no longer an issue between you and God under this new covenant of grace. The Bible says, "Neither by the blood of goats and calves, but by his own blood he entered in once into the holy place, having obtained eternal redemption for us" (Heb. 9:12). Eternal is forever and the word *redemption* means "forgiveness of sins." You are forgiven of your sin forever under the new covenant of grace. I am not condoning sin. Stay out of sin because it will open the door for the devil to attack you. Also, sin hurts people. I just want you to know that in God's eyes, he sees you in his Son. He sees you as being righteous.

Now let's talk about spirit, soul, and body again. God does not relate to you according to your flesh and the deeds of the flesh. God will never deal with your flesh (physical part of you). God will always see you as being in right standing with him because God is a spirit, and he is relating only to the spirit part of you. The Bible says, "God is a Spirit: and they that worship him must worship him in spirit and in truth" (John 4:24).

This is so important because so many Christians believe that they can't receive their healing or anything else because they are so unworthy because of the things they have done in the past. Christian people are always trying to measure up to some standard in order to receive from God or to be blessed by God. Most Christians believe that God is measuring them based on how good they are. They feel they have to qualify in some way to receive anything from God. They are trying to do what Jesus has already done for them. The truth is, we can never measure up to God's standard, that's why we needed a Savior, that's why we needed Jesus, and through him, we can measure up to God's standard. God is only responding to you based on what Jesus has already done for you and not what you can do for him. That's the grace of God. Believe that you are righteous now, and this will position you to take your healing.

Because you are righteous, you can say, "I have a blood brought right to be healed because I am the righteousness of God in Christ Jesus, and my right standing with God entitles me to divine health all my days on this earth." Your covenant of grace through Jesus Christ entitles you to be a covenant practitioner, and you now can respond to God for your healing based on your covenant. Glory to God!

You Must Get Rid of Fear

If you have been given a death sentence by a doctor, more than likely, you are very fearful.

You must get rid of fear because fear is contaminated faith. The world says a little fear is normal, but for the Christian, not only is fear not normal, it can't be tolerated on any level. You must not fear! Jesus said, "For God hath not given us the spirit of fear; but of power, and of love, and of a sound mind" (2 Tim. 1:7, KJV).

Jesus called fear a spirit and said if you are fearing, it doesn't come from him because he has given you power, love, and a sound mind. Jesus has given you power to overcome fear, and when you know how much he loves you, your mind will now become sound. Fear doesn't come from a sound mind or a mind that is fix on God and his Word. Fear comes from the devil! Fear contaminates your faith. Fear is contaminated faith. To get rid of fear, you must convince yourself of how much Jesus loves you, and that he won't let anything happen to you. To do this, you must confess over and over again: "God loves me, therefore, he is not going to let anything happen to me." As you say this over and over again, you will start to believe it, and fear will start to leave you. That's what the Bible mean when it says, "There is no fear in love; but perfect love casteth out fear: because fear hath torment. He that feareth is not made perfect in love" (1 John 4:18, KJV). If you are in fear, it's because you have not convinced yourself of how much God really loves you. When you are convinced of God's love for you, then that is perfect love, and it will cast out the fear.

You must convince yourself of this. You must put your trust totally in Jesus and believe that he is right there with you in this trial and that he will not let anything happen to you.

You Have Authority Over Sickness and Disease

The word authority means "the right to command". God has given you the right to command on the earth. The bible says "then God said, let us make man in our image, according to Our likeness; let them have dominion over the fish of the sea, over the birds of the air, and over the cattle, over all the earth and over every creeping thing that creeps on the earth." (Genesis 1:26) When God spoke these words he relinquished his authority in the earth to you "mankind". God no longer has authority, the right to command on the earth but you do. God can't do anything in the earth unless he does it through a physical man. God gave us the right to command in the earth. Notice the scriptures in Genesis 1:26 says you have authority (right to command) over all the earth. That word "all" means "all" Glory to God!

Anything in the earth that is not right you can use your authority to change it. Authority is released by speaking words. You must put the word of God in your mouth and speak it. Jesus himself says "For assuredly, I say to you, whosoever <u>says</u> to this mountain, be removed and be cast into the sea and does not doubt in his heart, but believers that those things he <u>says</u> will be done, he will have whatever he <u>says</u> (Mark 11:23). Notice Jesus says you have to speak to the mountain. You must speak to pain and tell it to leave your body. You must speak to "cancer" and tell it to leave your body. You might think to do this is silly but Jesus says to "speak to the mountain" this is how faith works. Jesus spoke to a fig tree and commanded it to die and it did. You speak to the pain and tell it to leave your body in Jesus name.

You speak to the disease (call it by name) and tell it to leave your body in Jesus name. You make the faith command in "Jesus name". What you are speaking to must obey the faith command when using the name of Jesus.

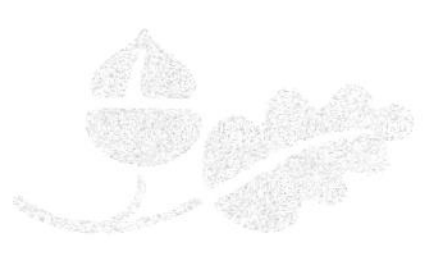

How the Kingdom of God Operates

Let's define the kingdom of God as being God's country and government on the inside of every born again believer. God's kingdom is independent of the world system. For example, when the stock market is crashing in the world, the kingdom of God is prospering. When the world system says, "We can treat it but there is no cure," God's kingdom says, "By His stripes you are already healed" (1 Pet. 2:24).

There are spiritual laws that govern the Kingdom of God but the Father of all the laws is the law of "Seedtime and Harvest". All spiritual laws are attached to this law. Everything in the Kingdom of God operates under this law. A seed is planted or sworn and a harvest manifest. The bible says, **Genesis 8:22 King James Version (KJV)**

> [22] While the earth remaineth, seedtime and harvest, and cold and heat, and summer and winter, and day and night shall not cease.

The law of Seedtime and Harvest is operating today. As you continue to read this book you will learn how to sow the seed of the word of God for healing into the ground of your heart and get it to produce in your life. The Kingdom that you have on the inside of you is very powerful! Apostle Paul said **1 Corinthians 4:20 King James Version (KJV)** [20] For the kingdom of God is not in word, but in power.

The Kingdom is very powerful and has everything you need to include healing. Jesus told the disciples[9] And heal the sick that are therein, and say unto them, The kingdom of God is come nigh unto you. The Kingdom released that healing power that healed them.

Why did Jesus say to tell them the Kingdom has come neigh unto them? The word neigh means "close" Kingdom came close to them. They were under the old covenant of the law and the Jesus hadn't died to give them the Kingdom, therefore, the Kingdom came neigh unto them. It is different for you the kingdom is inside of you in your spirit. The bible says, **Luke 17:20-21 King James Version (KJV)** [20]And when he was demanded of the Pharisees, when the kingdom of God should come, he answered them and said, The kingdom of God cometh not with observation: [21]Neither shall they say, Lo here! or, lo there! for, behold, the kingdom of God is within you.

The Kingdom has healing in it and is on the inside of you and you must get the kingdom to release the healing that you need.

You must believe the following truth:

1. You must believe that the kingdom does exist on the inside of you, and that healing is in the kingdom.
2. You must recognize that the Word of God (Scriptures) are spiritual laws designed to operate in the kingdom of God.
3. You must understand that the kingdom of God operates by the law of seedtime and harvest.
4. You must understand that the kingdom of God operates by principles.
5. You must understand that it pleases and glorifies the Father when we operate effectively in the kingdom and get results.

Most Christians have been taught that they don't need to do anything but trust God for what they need. This is not the entire truth. Yes, you must trust Jesus that healing has already been done; therefore, you are not asking God to heal you, healing is done. God is not making healing just because you need it, healing is done. Grace (God's undeserved favor) has made healing available, but you must take the healing with faith. In the covenant of grace, Jesus has done everything. The Bible says, "That ye be not slothful, but followers of them who through faith and patience inherit the promises" (Heb. 6:12).

The word *slothful* means "lazy." Christians today have been taught that everything that happens to them is in God's hand. Because they believe this, it has made them lazy and passive in exerting their faith. They believe that if they get healed, it is in God's hand and God's timing. I have heard this so much in religious circles. This is not true, whether you get healed or not is not in God's hand because he is not in control of your life and what happens to you but you are. The Bible says, "Submit yourselves therefore to God. Resist the devil, and he will flee from you" (James 4:7). This is a command from God himself. The sickness that you are experiencing is from Satan, so you must resist it. I will show you how to do that a little later in this book. God will not resist Satan for you, that is your part. God has done his part by providing healing by grace, but you must take it through faith.

All of the promises in the New Testament and all of the blessings in the Old Testament in Deuteronomy 28:1–14 belongs to you because you are under the covenant of grace that Jesus established with the Father on the cross. One of those promises or I can say one of the well-defined terms of the grace covenant is: "Who his own self bare our sins in his own body on the tree, that we, being dead to sins, should live unto righteousness: by whose stripes *ye were healed*" (1 Pet. 2:24). This promise belongs to you, but it won't just come on you automatically, you will never see the manifestation of it on your body without responding with faith. There has to be some action on your part, and that action is called faith.

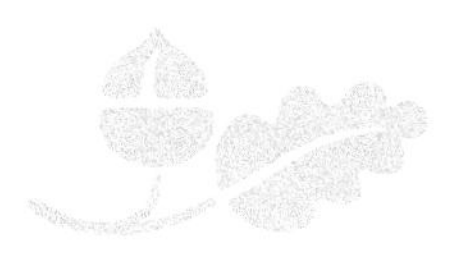

Steps to Taking Your Healing

Now let's look at the steps in obtaining your healing!

Step 1: You Must Speak to the Mountain

There is another law in the kingdom of God that you must cooperate with in getting healing to come to you, and that's the law that governs faith in the kingdom of God. This spiritual law says,

> And Jesus answering saith unto them, Have faith in God. For verily I say unto you, That whosoever shall say unto this mountain, Be thou removed, and be thou cast into the sea; and shall not doubt in his heart, but shall believe that those things which he saith shall come to pass; he shall have whatsoever he saith. Therefore I say unto you, What things soever ye desire, when ye pray, believe that ye receive them, and ye shall have them. (Mark 11:22–24, KJV)

This spiritual law says that you *must* speak to the mountain. The mountain in your life is the sickness that Satan is oppressing you with. Speak to it and tell it to leave your body. You must make this command in the name of Jesus. You may think this is silly, but remember Jesus spoke to the fig tree and cursed it. Everything in this earth is made to obey you when you speak to it in the name of Jesus. The thing is, not obeying you because you are speaking to it, but it has to obey you because of the name of Jesus that you are using. You have authority to use the name of Jesus, and you have authority over that disease. God gave you the authority in Genesis 1:26 (KJV): "And God said, Let us make man in our image, after our likeness: and let them have dominion over the fish of the sea, and over the fowl of the air, and over the cattle, and over all the earth, and over every creeping thing that creepeth upon the earth."

Cancer and any other disease is of the earth. You have authority over all the earth! Your mouth is the faucet that releases your authority. Your mouth is the faucet that releases your faith.

Now, let me show you how to speak to the mountain. For example, let's say cancer is the mountain. Do not do this in a passive attitude. You must let the devil know you mean business, so you must say this with authority. Say: "Cancer, I rebuke you in the name of Jesus, and you leave my body right now. You can't stay and you have no right to live in my body. You go now in Jesus's name!" Now a lot is happening in the spirit realm. That disease now has to obey the command given in Jesus's Name.

Every day, several times during the day, you speak to that cancer and say, "Cancer, you can't kill me. I will live and not die and declare the works of the Lord." That cancer is slowly dying because of the pressure that you are putting on it with the Word of God and your authority. You can do this with any disease.

Step 2: You Must Believe in Your Heart

The Scriptures are spiritual laws that work in the kingdom of God, and they can't be broken.

The Bible says,

> And Jesus answering saith unto them, Have faith in God. For verily I say unto you, That whosoever shall say unto this mountain, Be thou removed, and be thou cast into the sea; and shall

> not doubt in his heart, but shall believe that those things which he saith shall come to pass; he shall have whatsoever he saith. Therefore I say unto you, What things soever ye desire, when ye pray, believe that ye receive them, and ye shall have them. (Mark 11:22–24, KJV)

These Scriptures are spiritual laws that govern how faith works in the kingdom of God. Jesus says one of the criteria's for getting the Word to produce in your life is "shall not doubt in your heart." That means you must believe in your heart. Remember, your heart is your spirit and your soul (mind) together. Your spirit believes the things of God, but your soul (mind) doesn't when it is not renewed with the Word of God.

The way you get your heart to believe is you must "*Sow the healing seed of the word of God into the ground of your heart.*"

The Word of God is seed. Jesus said, "Now the parable is this: The seed is the word of God" (Luke 8:11, KJV).

You must think of the Scriptures as seed that you must sow in the ground of your heart to get it to manifest in your life. Let's think about something, if a farmer in the natural wants corn, he goes to the seed store and buy corn seed. He put the seed in the ground and water it, keep the weeds out, and eventually he will have corn. Well, you do the same thing in the spirit realm when you plant word *seed* and water it, keep the weeds out, and it will grow in your life. You don't go get any type of seed, you must get healing seed and plant it in the ground of your heart. For example, you get *1 Peter 2:24* and *Isaiah 53:4–5.* There are other healing seed as well. You must get specific seed because the seed produces after its own kind. An apple seed will produce only apples; therefore, healing seed will produce only healing.

Confessing the word will help you to believe in your heart. Another spiritual law is 2 Corinthians 4:13 (KJV): " We having the same spirit of faith, according as it is written, I believed, and therefore have I spoken; we also believe, and therefore speak." This spiritual law says whatever you say over and over and over again, you will start to believe. Therefore, when you first start to confess the healing Scriptures, your mind won't believe them because it is not renewed in the area of healing. Therefore, the more you confess the healing Scriptures, your mind will start to believe them. This is how you get your heart to believe. You must believe with all your heart. You are confessing the scriptures to believe that healing is on the inside of you. You must be fully persuaded.

There is reciprocal to every truth; therefore, if you are speaking the bad report of the doctor to everybody over and over and over again or if you are constantly talking about the pain and discomfort, you will start to believe that, and it will produce more and more in your life. What you speak, you believe; and what you believe, you will become. It's spiritual law!

Jesus tells us exactly how the Word of God can be planted into our heart and produce in our life.

> And he said, So is the kingdom of God, as if a man should cast seed into the ground; And should sleep, and rise night and day, and the seed should spring and grow up, he knoweth not how. For the earth bringeth forth fruit of herself; first the blade, then the ear, after that the full corn in the ear. (Mark 4:26–28, KJV)

Jesus says a man, not God, has to cast the seed of the Word of God into his heart. God will not cast the word *seed* into your heart for you. That's your part of the covenant to do. This is how you cooperate with spiritual laws. This is how you release your faith by speaking.

How do you cast seed into the ground of your heart?

You cast seed into the ground of your heart by:

1. Confessing healing scriptures aloud
2. Listening to healing scriptures on cd

3. Reading Jesus healing stories aloud in Mark, Luke, John and Matthew
4. Praising God and thanking him that you are healed before you see healing on your body

Your ears, eyes and mouth are the three gates to your heart (soul/spirit). These three are the avenues to which God word can enter into your heart (soul/spirit).

Start sowing healing seed into the ground of your heart. Once the seed is received in your heart (soul/spirit) it will start to release healing power on the inside of you. The more you speak the word, hear the word the seed is being watered and your spirit will put pressure on the word you are putting on the inside and you and cause it to grow and manifest on your physical body.

Watch You Mouth!

In teaching divine healing, I've seen where people are constantly talking about the different doctors they are going to and the different medicines they are taking. They are constantly talking about the doctors and the medicines. Thank God for the doctors and the medicines, and we need to work with the doctors and take the medicines because there is no wrong way of being healed as long as you get healed. But when you are talking about the doctors and the medicines more than the Word of God, then it creates unbelief in your heart. You are truly depending on the doctor and the medicine first instead of God and his Word.

So speak what the Word says about your healing over and over again until you believe it. As you do this, you will start to see yourself healed on the inside. How can this be? We see in pictures, not in words. If I said the word *dog*, you would see a picture of a dog in your mind. You would not see the word *dog* in your mind. Well, as you confess the healing Scriptures over and over and over again, the word you are confessing will paint a picture on the inside of you, and you will start to believe you are healed in spite of how you feel or the bad report of the doctor. As you confess the healing

Scriptures over and over again, you will persuade yourself of healing to such a degree that you won't even believe the bad report any more. You will start to believe beyond what your five senses (feel, taste, see, hear, and smell) reveals. You will believe you are healed beyond the contrary reports and what is happening in the natural. You will start to talk like you are healed, act like you are healed, and think that you are healed. No one will be able to convince you otherwise. You would be so convinced that you are healed because of the time you have invested in meditating and speaking healing word *seed* into the ground of your heart and painting a picture of healing on the inside of you. This is believing in the heart. Glory to God!

Step 3: You Must Get God's Faith to Come to You

God is a faith God! The Bible says, "But without faith it is impossible to please him: for he that cometh to God must believe that he is, and that he is a rewarder of them that diligently seek him" (Heb. 11:6, KJV). Without faith, God is not pleased because God knows that everything that Jesus Christ has already provided for you by grace (unearned favor) can only be obtained through faith. When you can't obtain your healing, God is not pleased.

The only way you can obtain the healing that grace has made available to you is through faith.

The Bible says, "By whom also *we have access by faith into this grace*_wherein we stand, and rejoice in hope of the glory of God" (Rom. 5:2, KJV). Faith is a creative force that causes things to appear. Faith is the only way to access healing that has been made available to you through grace.

You probably heard in the past that faith moves God. In the covenant of grace under the New Testament, faith is defined as "our positive response to what grace has made available." God is not making healing because you need it. God released his healing power for every man that will ever need healing two thousand years ago through Jesus. God's grace is the same to every man.

The Bible says, "Now faith is the substance of things hoped for, the evidence of things not seen" (Heb. 11:1, KJV). Faith gives substance to the thing that you are hoping for, which in this case is healing. Faith gives substance to healing. You can't see healing right now because it's in your spirit, but faith give substance to that healing, which means faith allows you to see the healing before it appears in the physical realm. Faith gives evidence to that which you can't see, smell, hear, feel, or taste. Faith gives evidence that the healing does exist beyond your five senses.

You need Bible faith to get the healing to come to you. You must understand that there are two types of faith. There is human faith or head faith. An example head faith is you walk into a room and you see a chair. You have faith that the chair will hold you, so you sat in it. Everyone is born with human or head faith. Another type of faith is God's faith or Bible faith. God's faith is the faith that is necessary to get healing to come to you. You can only get God's faith from the Scriptures. To get faith to come, you must confess the healing Scriptures, continuously believing that God's healing power is in those Scriptures. Other methods of getting God's faith to come to you is by listening to healing Scriptures on CDs, reading books on healing, to include the books of Mark, Luke, John, and Matthew aloud. Doing these things will cause you to be submerged in healing, and you will start to believe that you are healed. Remember, you can't have faith for something that you don't believe. You must first believe and then act on what you believe.

All the healing stories in the Bible where Jesus healed people, Jesus always said, "Your faith has made you whole." It was faith that was responsible for them getting healed, and it's faith that will be responsible for you receiving your healing as well.

Confessing the Scriptures over and over and over again, you are participating in the law of 2 Corinthians 4:13 (KJV): "We having the same spirit of faith, according as it is written, *I believed, and therefore have I spoken;* we also believe, and therefore speak."

This law simply says whatever you say over and over and over again, you will start to believe. This is why confessing the healing Scriptures continuously is so important. When you first start to confess them, you won't believe them; but as you continue to confess them, you will start to believe them. It's spiritual law! There is a reciprocal to every truth. If you confess doubt, fear, and unbelief continuously, you will start to believe that as well. If you are continuously talking about the bad doctor report, the pain, and symptoms that you feel, you will start to believe that, and it will increase in your life. So speak faith!

Confessing the healing Scriptures will allow you to see yourself healed on the inside before you ever see healing on the outside. Confessing the healing Scriptures will also renew your mind with healing and cause you to believe in your mind that you are healed. You will say, "I am healed" even when the doctor's x-ray show differently. You will just know on the inside that you are healed. You will become fully persuaded that you are healed before you ever see healing on your physical body. You will start to think that you are healed, act like you are healed, and talk like you are healed. This is evidence that you are now believing the Word of God, that you have been putting on the inside of you despite what you are seeing and hearing in the natural. The healing is taking place in the spirit part of you.

You are confessing the Word of God to believe it but also to get God's faith to come to you. God's faith is stored in his Scriptures; therefore, as you put those Scriptures in your eyes, speak them out of your mouth, and hear them in your ears, God's faith is being deposited on the inside of you through your soul (mind) and then deposited in your spirit. You are also cooperating with the spiritual law of Romans 10:17 (KJV) "So then faith cometh by hearing, and hearing by the word of God."

Your spirit man has a set of ears that pick up the words that you speak and send those words to your soul (mind) and then to your spirit. By confessing the healing Scriptures, God's faith that's in those Scriptures are being deposited on the inside of you. Once you are full of God's faith, your spirit will put pressure on the Word of God on the inside of you and cause the word to produce in your life. This is how God designed the Word to work on the inside of you. You must plant the seed of God's Word into your heart (soul/spirit) to get the word to manifest in your life

You may not totally understand sowing the seed of God's Word into your heart. It's okay because Jesus said you won't understand it. In the parable of the sower, Jesus tells us how to plant word seed into the ground of our heart and get it to produce in our lives. "And he said, So is the kingdom of God, as if a man should cast seed into the ground; And should sleep, and rise night and day, and the seed should spring and grow up, he knoweth not how" Mark 4:26–27 (KJV). All you need to do is put the Word of God into your heart and get faith to come to you. The force of faith will cause it to produce in your life.

To get God's faith, you must find the specific healing Scriptures in the Bible, put them in your eyes, speak them out your mouth, and when you do this, you are sowing word seed into the ground of your heart. You have the garden of Eden on the inside of you in your spirit. When you speak healing Scriptures out of your mouth, you are cooperating with spiritual laws.

The Scriptures are laws that operate in the kingdom of God on the inside of you. You must cooperate with those laws to get the Word of God to manifest in your life. The law that governs faith in the kingdom of God is *Mark 11:23 (KJV)*:

> For verily I say unto you, That whosoever shall say unto this mountain, Be thou removed, and be thou cast into the sea; and shall not doubt in his heart, but shall believe that those things which he saith shall come to pass; he shall have whatsoever he saith.

God has stored his faith in the Scriptures, so when you confess (declare and speak) out of your mouth what God has said about your healing, God's faith is going into your soul (mind) and renewing it to the fact that healing exist on the inside of you. Confessing the Scriptures not only get rid of doubt in the soul (mind), it puts God's faith into your heart. Glory to God!

Step 4: Your Faith Must Not Be Passive

The word *passive* in the dictionary means "accepting or allowing what happens or what others do without active response or resistance." The Bible says, "Submit yourselves therefore to God. *Resist the devil, and he will flee from you*" (James 4:7, KJV). This is your part of the covenant. You must resist the devil, and he'll flee from you. God will not resist the devil for you.

In teaching divine healing from a grace perspective, I've noticed that often time people's faith (action and words) are very passive. When teaching them how to cooperate with the spiritual laws to get healing to come to them, they are very passive in acting on what they are taught. They don't do it with aggressiveness being totally focus on getting the healing to come to them, and as a result, they don't obtain the healing. The Bible says, "And from the days of John the Baptist until now the kingdom of heaven suffereth violence, and the violent take it by force" (Matt. 11:12, KJV). Although healing belongs to you and is your covenant right, you will have to take the healing by enforcing these spiritual laws. You will have to possess the healing. Everything you get from the kingdom you will have to possess because Satan will fight you.

Satan is trying to take the healing that Jesus has already given you. Remember, the children of Israel had to possess the land even though it belonged to them. God had already given it to them, but they had to possess it. To possess means to take ownership of something. You will have to release violent faith to take your healing. Every person in the Bible that received healing from Jesus had violent faith. They were not passive in their faith. In *Mark chapter 10*, blind Bartimaeus, when he heard that Jesus was passing by, started releasing his faith by shouting and making so much noise that the religious folk around him told him to be quiet, but the Bible says he didn't care what the people around him thought, he was desperate to receive his sight, so the more they told him to be quiet, the louder he got. This is radical faith. It is something about being desperate that gets the healing. He was so persistent with his faith, and as a result, he got the attention of Jesus. Violent faith gets the attention of Jesus!

The four men in *Luke chapter 5* that peeled off the roof of the house that Jesus was having a meeting in and lowered their friend down so Jesus could heal him had violent faith. Jesus told them that their faith had healed the man. Passive faith will not get the attention of Jesus. The woman with the issue of blood in *Mark chapter 5* came behind Jesus and took her healing. She placed a demand on the healing anointing that was in his garment. She took it!

I think what has contributed to Christian people being so passive in acting on the Word of God where healing is concern is the fact that religion has dumbed so many Christians down to think that if God wants them healed, then he would just heal them or God doesn't heal everybody. God has released his healing power by his grace for anyone that will need it.

Another contributor to Christians having passive faith is the sovereignty of God teaching, which states that God is totally in control of everything that happens whether good or bad, and if you are sick, then it must be God's will. God is not in control of everything he has given control of the earth to man (Gen. 1:26). If you think that it is God's will for you to be sick, then you won't contend for your healing because you will think that you are fighting against God. This makes your faith very passive. If it is God's will for you to be sick, then why pray or go to the doctor? Why do anything if it is God's will that you be sick? Why take medicine if it is God's will that you be sick? God is not in control of our lives, we are. This teaching makes Christians think that their getting healed is all in God's hand, and they don't have a part to play in them receiving their healing. They are in covenant with God through Jesus Christ, and healing is in the covenant. They must realize that when they cooperate with spiritual laws of the covenant, the healing power is released.

The Bible says, "My son, attend to my words; incline thine ear unto my sayings. Let them not depart from thine eyes; keep them in the midst of thine heart. For they are life unto those that find them, and health to all their flesh" (Prov. 4:20–22, KJV).

To attend to the Word means to focus on the Word, make it a priority talk about it more than anything else. You must incline your ears to what God's Word has already said about your healing. Speak

God's Word about healing out of your mouth constantly and hear it constantly so you can believe it so faith can come to you. Don't keep rehearsing the bad doctor report. Tell people that you are healed. You may say, "Well, I feel like am lying if I do that." How can you be lying, saying what God has already said about your healing? You will be speaking the solution, not the problem. Notice *verse 22* says that the Word of God is life and health to all your flesh. The word *health* in the Hebrew is translated "medicine." The Word of God is medicine to your body so take the medicine. Glory to God!

Every time you quote the healing Scriptures and listen to them on CDs or read healing stories, you are sowing healing seed into the ground of your heart. This is how the kingdom operate. The Word on the inside of you starts to release its power and gradually destroy that disease from the inside of you.

If you are dealing with a terminal disease, you must realize that the disease is working twenty-four hours a day to kill you; therefore, your works of faith must be aggressive and working on that same level to destroy that disease.

What is the works of faith? Confessing healing Scriptures, listening to healing scriptures on CDs, reading the book of Mark, Luke, John, and Matthew aloud to yourself. These books contain the healing stories of Jesus in them, and when you read them aloud, Jesus faith for healing that in those Scriptures are coming on the inside of you. You should play the healing Scriptures on CD all night long very softly while you are sleeping. Purchase a CD player with a repeat-all feature on it. Remember, your soul and spirit can receive while you are sleeping. This is how you resist the devil. ***Submerge yourself in healing*** and watch God's healing power destroy that disease. Glory to God!

You must constantly act like you are healed, talk like you are healed, and think like you are healed. Don't talk how you feel in your physical body. Don't talk about the pain, instead speak to the pain. Speak to the mountain, and tell the pain to leave your body in Jesus's name!

As you renew your mind to healing, all these things will become natural for you to do.

You must not accept a bad report from the doctor. Well, Sonja, what should I say if the doctor says, "We can treat it but there is no cure"? If you can't speak faith, don't say anything. Don't agree with the bad report. Just be quiet. Remember, your words set the course as to how this situation is going to turn out. Once you get in your car, just say, "Father, you heard the bad report from the doctor, but I don't receive it, instead I believe what you said about my healing in *1 Peter 2:24*, and I believe I receive my healing right now by the stripes of Jesus. Thank you." Now start working the works of faith!

Most Christians don't want to do this because they are concern as to what people will think about them. But when you are fighting for your life, you must be like blind Bartemaeus who didn't consider the people around him because he wanted his healing. You must saturate yourself in healing. Read books on healing. Look at healing teaching from past evangelist such as Oral Roberts, Gloria Copeland healing school and Andrew Wommack *Healing Is Here* conference and *God Wants You Well* teaching series. Also listen to Youtube healing teachings by Sonja Parham. Type "Sonja Parham" in the Youtube browser. Kenneth Hagan healing school, and many others. These teachings can be found on YouTube. Saturate yourself in them instead of watching television. This will build your faith for healing.

It's faith that gives substance to healing according to *Hebrews 11:1*. Its violent faith that gets you whole (healed). I talk to so many people that say, "I'm praying for God to heal me." There is a time to pray and there is a time to take your authority over the situation. Prayer alone didn't get any of the people in the Bible healed. Jesus said it was their faith that made them whole, not prayer. They had to do something as an act of faith to respond to the healing anointing that Jesus was anointed with. You will have to respond to Jesus (who is in Word form). You will have to respond to the Word of God to take your healing. You must mix faith with the Word of God, and faith is always in action and words. It's your faith that will make you whole.

Step 5: You Must Release Faith

Faith is released in two ways, through words and action.

The faith that you are releasing is God's faith. You are operating in God's faith, not yours. The Bible says, "Looking unto Jesus the author and finisher of our faith; who for the joy that was set before him endured the cross, despising the shame, and is set down at the right hand of the throne of God" (Heb. 12:2 KJV). Jesus has given you his supernatural faith that is in his Word.

Now, you must release that faith. Let's talk about how to release faith to get the healing to come to you. You release faith when you cooperate with God's spiritual laws.

You must understand that the Scriptures are spiritual laws that were established by God, and when you cooperate with them, then they cause the Word of God to manifest in your life. Cooperating with spiritual laws are the way you release faith. The Bible says, "Even so faith, if it hath not works, is dead, being alone" (James 2:17, KJV). You must release corresponding action to what you believe, and this is called faith. Let's look at the spiritual laws you must cooperate with and how to do it. The first law is the law of calling things that be not as though they were.

> [As it is written, I have made thee a father of many nations,] before him whom he believed, even God, who quickeneth the dead, and *calleth those things which be not as though they were.* (Rom. 4:17, KJV)

God used the law of calling things that be not as though they were in calling Abraham a father of many nations before he even had a child.

You must call yourself healed before you even see the healing on your physical body. Don't say "I'm sick," but say, "I'm healed by the stripes of Jesus." Don't say what you see in the natural but what you see in the spirit, in God's Word. Tell people you are healed. Don't tell them that you are sick. Call the healing that be not as though it were. Glory to God!

The second law is the law of *what you believe you speak and what you speak you believe*. The Apostle Paul said in 2 Corinthians 4:13 (KJV), "We having the same spirit of faith, according as it is written, *I believed, and therefore have I spoken*; we also believe, and therefore speak." This spiritual law says that what you say over and over and over again you will start to believe. Say what God has said about your healing from the Bible.

Step 6: Don't Choke the Seed

The Word of God is seed that you must plant in the ground of your heart. When you are doing the things that we just discussed earlier, you are putting healing word seed on the inside of you. The Bible says, "Now the parable is this: The seed is the word of God" (Luke 8:11, KJV).

You must plant spiritual word *seed* the same way you plant a natural seed. If you plant corn seed in the ground, you must water it and pull out all the weeds that will keep it from growing. Well, you must keep weeds out of the ground of your heart when you are planting healing seed. You don't want the weeds to choke the healing seed that you are putting inside of you and keep it from growing. You may be asking, "What are the weeds that can choke the seed?" The weeds are religion, traditions of men, all the unbelief on television and social media. When you are in a fight for your life, doctor has diagnosed you with a terminal disease, it is not the time to be watching television. *Get_away from the television,* all the things you hear and see on television is unbelief, and it will choke the healing seed on the inside of you. Keep healing seed on the inside of you, and it will produce on your physical body.

Don't choke the healing seed that you are putting on the inside of you with negative words.

Watch the words that you are speaking, and make sure they are words of faith, not words of doubt and unbelief.

Step 7: Walk in Love

God has given the New Testament Christian one commandment. The bible say "a new commandment I give unto you. That ye love one another, as I have loved you that ye also love one another (John 13:34). Everything in the Kingdom of God operates from the platform of love, therefore, you must stay out of strife (arguments with people) and walk in unconditional love while you are waiting for your healing to manifest. Strife can stop the healing from flowing to you. Bitterness and unforgiveness are anointing blockers also. These issues can stop you from receiving your healing so make sure these issues are not in your heart.

Healing Is a Process

When you start doing all the things you have learned in this book continuously, on a daily basis, you might not see any physical change in your body right away because divine healing is a gradual process. You may have symptoms of sickness on your body for a while, but know that the healing is taking place in your spirit and will gradually come on the outside of you. Remember, Jesus cursed the fig tree, and it was hours later that they saw that it had dried up from the roots. The dying process started under the ground and physical evidence was seen above ground hours later. This is how things work in the spirit realm. Healing starts in your spirit where you can't see or feel it. Jesus gives us a perfect illustration of how the Word produces in our lives in Mark 4:26–28 (KJV),

> And he said, So is the kingdom of God, as if a man should cast seed into the ground; And should sleep, and rise night and day, and the seed should spring and grow up, he knoweth not how. For the earth bringeth forth fruit of herself; *first the blade, then the ear, after that the full corn in the ear.*

Notice Jesus said that the corn itself doesn't produce immediately but the blade, then the ear, and after that, the full corn. The kingdom process, in most cases, is a gradual process. In light of this, you just get up every morning and do all that you have learned in this book continuously everyday over and over and over again and go to sleep and do it the next day and the next day until the healing manifest on your physical body.

Make Your Body Respond

Often times when our physical body is experiencing symptoms of sickness and disease, we want to respond to the body by doing what it want. The body want to lay in the bed all day and talk about how it feels. You must resist your body and what it wants to do. Do something that you couldn't do before. Everyday do something that you couldn't do on yesterday. I remember once I had symptoms of the flu and I was standing on the word of God for my healing, but I was laying in the bed most of the day. The Lord said to me "healed people don't lay in bed all day." I immediately got up and started to do my housework and within a matter of a few hours all my symptoms were gone. Glory to God!

Receive Your Healing

It's not enough to take (possess) your healing you must receive it. You now know how to possess (take) healing by cooperating with spiritual laws of the Kingdom. You must not do these things religiously or mechanically, but do them knowing that you are simply releasing your faith for your healing. There is a difference between taking your healing and receiving it. Receiving happens in the heart (soul/spirit).

Let me give you an example of what I am talking about. If you saw a box wrapped in beautiful wrapping paper with a gift on the inside of it in a chair and you walked over and took the box you now possess it because it's in your hand. Although you have possession of the box the gift doesn't do you any good until you receive it by opening the box. Opening the box is how you receive the gift. Therefore, it is possible to possess something and not experience it because you never received it. It is the same way with faith. You take (possess) your healing by doing all the faith steps discussed previously but now you have to receive your healing. Receiving happens on the inside of you in your heart (soul/spirit). You must understand that your healing is a reality in the spirit realm and you doing all the steps to take your healing is born out of your belief and not your works. In other words, if you truly believe everything you have read in this book you will now respond to what you believe with action. To take your healing you must believe that you are healed right now in spite of what you are experiencing in your body. In the covenant of grace everything is done and you simply take Jesus at his word when he says you are already healed (1 Peter 2:24). When you are fully persuaded and have full confidence on the inside of you that you are healed no matter what you see or what is said that's when you have received your healing. Evidence that you have received your healing in your heart (soul/spirit) is when things are getting worse and you say "I don't care how things look Jesus has already healed me" that's when the healing has been received. When you are totally depending upon Jesus and you know that Jesus purchased your healing and has given it to you as a gift healing will flow to you. You must trust in Jesus for your healing and not you doing something to get healed. Jesus has already done it for you by his grace.

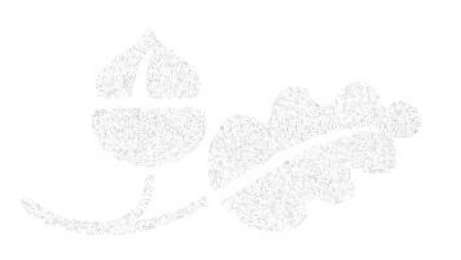

How to Maintain Your Healing Once You Receive It

Once healing has manifested on your physical body, there are some things you must do to maintain that healing. Katherine Khulman was a powerful healing evangelist. Records revealed that God worked mightily in her healing meetings. People were healed of all kinds of sicknesses and diseases. I once heard a well-known evangelist that worked in her meetings say that he heard her say that 90 percent of the people that were healed in her meetings, the diseases came back on them within one year. The reason for this is because they all were healed on her anointing and not on their faith in the Word of God. When you are healed on someone else anointing, there is the possibility that Satan can steal that healing because you don't really have understanding of healing, but when you are healed with your own faith standing on the Word of God with understanding, Satan can't steal that healing because you understand how you got healed. Jesus said in Matthew 13:19 (KJV), "When any one heareth the word of the kingdom, and understandeth it not, then cometh the wicked one, and catcheth away that which was sown in his heart. This is he which received seed by the way side." The Word of the kingdom is the Scriptures in the Bible. Jesus said, if you don't have understanding of what you are doing with the Scriptures, then Satan can take the Word from you. This is why teaching the Word of God and how to use it is vital to Christians in these last days. You must understand how to use the Word of God to get the kingdom to produce what you need in your life. This is why this book was written, to give you understanding of how to use the Word of God to take your healing.

To maintain your healing, you must keep enough of the Word of God where healing is concern on the inside of you; therefore, you must always every day until you leave this earth meditate on the healing Scriptures. You can take the time before you go to bed at night or when you rise early in the morning. You must keep healing seed on the inside of you.

Another thing that is helpful in maintaining your healing is to attend a church that teaches healing. If you attend a religious church that doesn't believe in healing and doesn't teach healing, then what you hear in that church could put unbelief in you and cause the healing to leave you. Jesus gave us a perfect example of this in Mark 8:22–24 (KJV):

> And he cometh to Bethsaida; and they bring a blind man unto him, and besought him to touch him. And he took the blind man by the hand, and led him out of the town; and when he had spit on his eyes, and put his hands upon him, he asked him if he saw ought. And he looked up, and said, I see men as trees, walking.

Notice Jesus had to take the man out of that city of unbelief in order to heal him. Unbelief will stop the healing anointing from flowing. An environment of unbelief on a continuous basis will also hinder you in maintaining your healing. Find a church that teaches the Word of God (Scriptures) and teaches healing.

To maintain your healing, you must stay out of sin. Although under the new covenant, your sins are forgiven. Your past, present, and future sin is no longer an issue between you and God; however, sin will open the door for the devil to put that disease back on you. Jesus tells us this in John 5:14 (KJV), "Afterward Jesus findeth him in the temple, and said unto him, Behold, thou art made whole: sin no more, lest a worse thing come unto thee."

After receiving his healing, Jesus tells the man if he get into sin that a worse thing may come upon him.

Hear and be healed! In conclusion you must not tolerate chronic pain or sickness and disease as they are works of the devil. Remember, what you tolerate today you will live with tomorrow. Don't tolerate pain or sickness and disease on any level. Take the word of God with your authority and drive that pain and disease out of your body.

If you need healing cards and healing Scriptures on CD, please contact:
Sonja Parham Ministries
P.O. Box 3622, Petersburg, Virginia 23805
Tel: (804) 919-1105, email: sonjapar@aol.com

About the Author

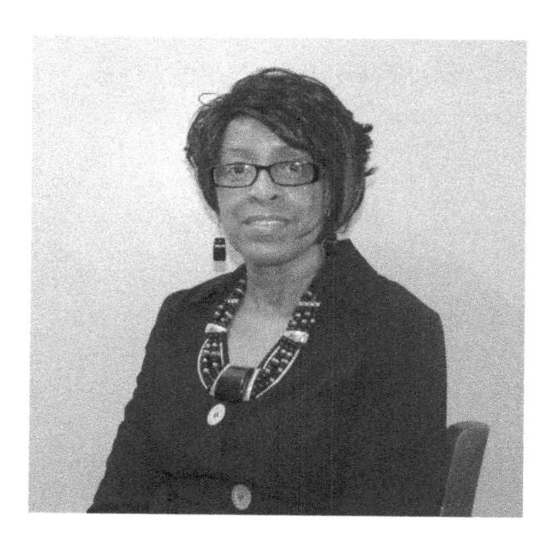

Sonja H. Parham is a grace preacher and teacher that believes Jesus has already done everything for the believer through his work on the cross at Calvary. Healing, prosperity, abundance, soundness, and wholeness in every area of the believer's life is already done by grace (God's undeserved favor).

Sonja hosts various healing and faith seminars. She is the founder of Sonja Parham Ministries, Inc.

She has a Bachelor of Science degree in business administration from Virginia State University and Certificates from Oral Roberts University School of The Spirit. Sonja is married with five children and six grandchildren.

CPSIA information can be obtained
at www.ICGtesting.com
Printed in the USA
BVHW031446150521
607358BV00007B/783